Navigating Life on Dialysis:
A Patient's Survival Guide

by Lord M. A. Daley Sr.

ISBN: 9798395040039
Imprint: Independently published

TABLE OF CONTENT.
Page

Chapter 1. Dialysis for Beginners
9
Chapter 2. Coping with the Emotional Impact of Dialysis
16
Chapter 3. Diet and Nutrition
21
Chapter 4. Managing Medication on Dialysis
27
Chapter 5. Exercise on Dialysis
33
Chapter 6. Dialysis Complications and How to Prevent Them
39
Chapter 7. Strategies for Dealing with Dialysis-Related
Fatigue
47
Chapter 8. Advocating for Yourself:
Tips for Communicating with Healthcare Providers   53
Chapter 9. Maintaining Relationships
59
Chapter 10. Life After Dialysis:

Preparing for a Kidney Transplant or End-of-Life Care   64

Bibliography
71
More about author
73

Chapter 1: Dialysis for Beginners

Chapter 1: Dialysis for Beginners

Let's dive right in with the basics of dialysis. Dialysis is an essential life-sustaining treatment for those living with kidney failure. Your kidneys are responsible for clearing out waste and excess fluid from your body. When they stop functioning correctly, dialysis becomes necessary to ensure this waste is removed from your body's system.

This guide is written specifically for those who have recently been diagnosed with kidney failure or about to start treatment and would like to understand more about dialysis treatment and its basics.

First, what is dialysis? Dialysis is a medical treatment that filters blood to get rid of extra fluid and waste products from the body, typically using a machine called dialysis machines to purge and cleanse blood for proper fluid and electrolyte balance in the body. Dialysis becomes necessary when kidneys no longer function normally due to disease, e.g., kidney failure or end-stage renal disease (ESRD).

Types of Dialysis

There are two major forms of dialysis treatment: haemodialysis and peritoneal dialysis.

Haemodialysis

Haemodialysis, also referred to as blood cleansing through machine and filter, involves extracting blood from the body and passing it through an electrolytic filter that removes waste products and excess fluid before returning it back into circulation. Haemodialysis sessions usually last four hours each and may be done in either a dialysis centre or home setting. The haemodialysis machine is connected to the body via a catheter, fistula, or a graft. But we will go deeper into this in just a minute.

Peritoneal Dialysis

Peritoneal dialysis is a procedure in which a special solution is used to purify blood. A catheter is inserted into the abdominal cavity, and this solution is pumped directly into it to absorb wastes and excess fluids, which then drain out of the body through drains. Peritoneal dialysis should typically be performed several times each day at home and should take between one to four hours per session.

Preparing for Dialysis

Dialysis requires careful preparation and planning. Before starting dialysis treatments, patients must undergo various tests to assess kidney function and overall health status, working closely with their physicians to ensure a smooth experience.

Preparing for Haemodialysis

Before beginning haemodialysis, patients must undergo a minor surgery to create either a fistula or graft. A fistula connects an artery and vein, while a graft uses artificial vessels to connect these organs. Both connections allow blood to move from your body and back in through a dialysis machine. You also must purchase equipment and supplies needed for dialysis at home.

Preparing for Peritoneal Dialysis

Before beginning peritoneal dialysis, a catheter must be implanted into the abdominal cavity, and patients should ensure they have the necessary supplies, such as dialysis solution, bags, and tubing.

After Dialysis

Following dialysis treatments, patients may become tired and weak. It is essential that patients stay hydrated by drinking sufficient fluids in order to avoid dehydration. Additionally, following a balanced diet can also help balance electrolytes. Furthermore, it is also beneficial for them to maintain a healthy lifestyle with regular exercise, checkups, and good sleeping habits.

Benefits and Risks of Dialysis Treatment

Dialysis offers many advantages for patients waiting for kidney transplants. Furthermore, dialysis treatment can enhance quality of life for people living with kidney failure by alleviating symptoms like fatigue, nausea, and swelling.

Dialysis does carry some risks. Infection at the site of catheter or graft placement could occur, and bleeding could take place during dialysis procedures. Furthermore, low blood pressure could result in dizziness, fainting, or even heart failure for some individuals.

Conclusion

Dialysis is a medical treatment designed to keep those living with kidney failure healthy and alive. Patients must go through several tests and preparation procedures prior to beginning dialysis treatment, which each has benefits and risks that they must discuss with healthcare providers. By understanding the basics of dialysis treatment, they can make informed decisions regarding their care plan while managing their condition effectively.

Chapter 2: Coping with the Emotional Impact of Dialysis

Chapter 2: Coping with the Emotional Impact of Dialysis

Diagnosing end-stage renal disease (ESRD) and beginning dialysis treatment is often an emotional journey for many patients. While dialysis treatment is necessary to survival, its emotional side effects may cause significant distress to patients who must continue dialysis treatment for prolonged periods. Coping with its impact is paramount to remaining well and continuing treatment successfully.

Patients on dialysis may encounter several emotional challenges, including anxiety, depression, fear, and frustration. Anxiety may arise due to its invasive nature and associated uncertainty regarding outcomes. Depression could follow due to loss of independence and physical limitations leading to sadness or hopelessness. Fear can surface from potential complications and whether treatment will ultimately succeed. Frustration stems from the time commitment required for dialysis as well as the restrictions it places on daily life.

One of the best ways to manage the emotional effects of dialysis is to recognise and express one's feelings. Patients shouldn't feel ashamed to talk about how dialysis has changed them or is overwhelming them. Support groups provide an excellent platform for sharing emotions while getting assistance in the form of counselling, social workers, or psychiatrists. If needed, talk to your renal team.

Another way to manage the emotional toll of dialysis is through exercise. While dialysis may limit some physical activities, patients can still find ways to stay active throughout their treatment plan, such as walking or stretching. Exercise releases endorphins that combat anxiety and depression for better psychological well-being.

You should also cultivate a positive outlook. Patients should concentrate on what they can control rather than dwelling on what cannot change. Having such an outlook will keep patients motivated and committed to their treatment, in a way guaranteeing the best possible results.

Stress management is imperative. While dialysis itself may be stressful, patients can use techniques like deep breathing and mindfulness to decrease stress levels. These practices bring peace and reduce anxiety levels significantly while improving overall mental health.

Attentiveness to one's emotional well-being while on dialysis is also key. Patients should pursue hobbies they find enjoyable, such as reading, painting, listening to music, or my favourite, playing video games, as ways of relieving stress and distracting themselves from dialysis' challenges. Hobbies can provide relief from anxiety and depression while contributing to overall better mental health.

Strong support systems can make an enormous difference. Family and friends can provide much-needed emotional and practical assistance, making managing dialysis much simpler.

Chapter 3: Diet and Nutrition

Chapter 3: Diet and Nutrition

Dialysis can be an invaluable lifeline for individuals living with end-stage renal disease (ESRD). Dialysis can have lasting impacts on your diet. Proper nutrition must be prioritised to ensure patients receive essential nutrients, maintain a healthy weight, and avoid malnutrition.

Diet and nutrition play an indisputable role in dialysis treatment. Patients must adhere to a stringent diet that limits sodium, potassium, phosphorus, fluid intake, and bone disorders that could result in serious health conditions like high blood pressure. They need to collaborate closely with a registered dietitian in creating a meal plan tailored to them and their unique dietary requirements.

One of the primary dietary goals for dialysis patients should be limiting their sodium consumption. Sodium can be found in many foods, and too much sodium can lead to fluid retention and increased blood pressure, potentially resulting in swelling. Dialysis patients may be advised to consume fresh fruit and vegetables, lean proteins, and limit the intake of processed food products that tend to be high in sodium content. It is also wise for dialysis patients to read nutrition labels closely when selecting low-sodium options.

Potassium is another essential nutrient for dialysis patients to monitor. Potassium can be found in foods such as bananas, oranges, potatoes, and tomatoes. Its levels in the body are controlled by kidneys. When your kidneys fail, potassium levels can build up, leading to heart issues. An individual's daily recommended potassium intake depends on their serum potassium levels and may differ depending on each person undergoing dialysis treatment.

Phosphorus, an essential mineral found in many food items like dairy products, meat, beans, and nuts, can become toxic when kidney function deteriorates and the toxics in the blood increase, leading to bone disorders and cardiovascular disease. Dialysis patients may be advised to limit their consumption of high-phosphorus foods and prescribed phosphate binders to prevent excessive absorption in their bodies.

Most find this next one a bit hard: fluid management. Dialysis patients should limit their fluid consumption to prevent an overload, which can lead to shortness of breath, high blood pressure, and fluid accumulation in the legs and other parts of the body. Dialysis patients are advised to maintain a record of their fluid consumption as well as receive specific restrictions depending on body weight and urine output.

Dialysis patients may be advised to supplement their nutrition with vitamins and minerals to meet their dietary needs, such as iron supplements for anaemia prevention and vitamin D or calcium supplements for bone health improvement. When considering any supplement regimens, patients should always consult their medical team beforehand as taking certain vitamins may interact negatively with medications they take.

Maintaining a healthy weight is of utmost importance for dialysis patients. Being over or underweight can have severe health repercussions, including heart disease, malnutrition, and poor wound healing. Working with a registered dietitian and engaging in regular physical activity are the two key ingredients necessary for reaching this goal.

Diet and nutrition play an essential role in managing dialysis patients. Adherence to a diet low in sodium, potassium, phosphorus, fluids, and fluid-borne calories as well as monitoring vitamin and mineral intake is critical in helping dialysis patients avoid health problems while improving quality of life. Dialysis patients must collaborate closely with their medical team and registered dietitian in creating an individualised meal plan tailored specifically for them; by adhering to healthy dietary recommendations while managing nutrient intake as well as weight control strategies they can live long fulfilling lives.

In conclusion, dialysis can be a lifeline for individuals with ESRD, but proper nutrition must be a priority to maintain overall health and wellbeing. Collaboration with a registered dietitian is critical in developing a tailored meal plan that prioritises essential nutrients while limiting sodium, potassium, and phosphorus intake. By adhering to this diet plan, patients can minimise the lasting impact of dialysis treatment on their overall health and quality of life.

Chapter 4: Managing Medication on Dialysis

Chapter 4: Managing Medication on Dialysis

Many ESRD patients require multiple medications in addition to dialysis treatments in order to manage symptoms and avoid complications. Properly dosing medications while on dialysis may prove challenging but must remain a top priority in order for patients to experience positive health outcomes.

Due to the complex nature of dialysis treatment, patients must utilise proper medication management strategies to receive effective therapy. Dialysis may alter how drugs are absorbed and eliminated from the body as well as change concentration levels in the blood. Therefore, it's crucial that dosages are carefully adjusted according to each patient's kidney function and dialysis regime.

Drug interactions pose another significant challenge to dialysis medication management. Dialysis patients frequently take multiple drugs to manage various conditions such as hypertension, diabetes, anaemia, and cardiovascular disease, but some interactions between medications could potentially cause adverse reactions or diminish effectiveness of therapies. As such, they must be closely monitored in order to avoid health complications and side effects.

Effective Strategies for Administering Dialysis Medication

Medication management on dialysis requires an integrative approach involving all parties involved: patient, healthcare team, and caregiver. Here are some strategies that may assist with optimising medication administration on dialysis:

1. Keep an Updated Medication List

Dialysis patients must remain aware of all their medications, including dosages, timing, and potential side effects. It is important that an updated medication list be shared with the healthcare team and caregiver so they can assist in monitoring medications and detect any discrepancies or irregularities that arise.

2. Collaborate with the Healthcare Team

Dialysis patients should maintain regular contact with their healthcare team, consisting of the primary care physician, nephrologist, pharmacist, and dietitian. These individuals can assist in managing medications and dosage adjustments as necessary, as well as provide advice about interactions, potential side effects, and lifestyle modifications that will maximise the efficacy of medications prescribed to them.

3. Stick to Your Medication Schedule

Dialysis patients must adhere to a regimented medication schedule in order to take their drugs at the prescribed times and in the right amounts, without missing doses or double-upping on medications which could result in dangerous drug interactions or toxicities. Pill organisers or alarms are essential reminders of medications times and should always be in use.

4. Be Alert for Adverse Side Effects

Dialysis patients should remain aware of possible side effects from medication used on dialysis and immediately inform their healthcare team if any adverse reactions arise, including nausea, dizziness, fatigue, or headaches that might indicate drug toxicity or overdose.

5. Be Wary of Over-the-Counter Medications

Dialysis patients should exercise extreme caution when taking over-the-counter medications, even though these might appear harmless. Unfortunately, however, they can interact with prescribed drugs, causing adverse side effects and diminishing treatment efficacy. It's best to consult your healthcare team first before making decisions.

Chapter 5: Exercise on Dialysis

Chapter 5: Exercise on Dialysis

Exercise and physical activity play an integral role in improving functional status, mitigating complications, and increasing quality of life, though exercise for dialysis patients must be conducted carefully due to unique challenges involved.

Regular exercise and physical activity have been demonstrated to offer many health advantages for dialysis patients, such as:

1. Improved Cardiovascular Function

Cardiovascular disease is a significant complication among dialysis patients, often associated with increased mortality rates. Regular exercise has been proven to enhance cardiovascular function, lower high blood pressure, and decrease the risk of heart disease.

2. Increased Strength and Endurance

Dialysis patients typically experience muscle fatigue from chronic kidney disease treatments, such as dialysis. Regular physical exercise can help strengthen muscles, increase endurance levels, and prevent frailty.

3. Improved Mental Health

Dialysis patients tend to experience elevated rates of depression and anxiety due to their chronic illnesses and related lifestyle restrictions, making daily life increasingly challenging. Regular physical activity has been proven to significantly decrease incidence and severity of depression, anxiety, and stress levels among these individuals.

4. Improved Bone Health

Dialysis patients face increased risks for osteoporosis and fractures as a result of bone density loss, but regular physical exercise can improve bone density, decrease fracture risk, and contribute to overall health benefits. Precautions to Consider for Exercise and Physical Activity While on Dialysis

Patients living with end-stage renal disease require special consideration and guidance when engaging in exercise to ensure safe and beneficial results. Here are a few key precautions:

1. Consult with a Healthcare Professional

Before initiating any exercise program, patients must always consult their healthcare provider first. Their doctor should assess their current state of health, medical history, and dialysis regimen in detail.

2. Begin Slowly and Gradually Increase

For best results, exercise should begin slowly with gradual increases in intensity and duration. Patients returning from an absence may begin with short walks or light exercises. Listening to your body and taking into consideration individual preferences are the keys to successful workouts.

3. Monitor Fluid Intake Dialysis patients must carefully manage their fluid intake. Excessive consumption during exercise can lead to fluid overload, which has serious repercussions for kidney health and should be prevented through consultation with their healthcare professional in creating an exercise-specific fluid management plan.

4. Monitor Blood Sugar Levels
Diabetes is an increasingly prevalent side effect of dialysis treatments, and exercise may alter the levels of blood glucose in dialysis patients. Individuals living with diabetes should monitor their blood glucose before and after participating in physical activities and adjust their insulin regimen as necessary.

5. Consider Physical Limitations
Dialysis patients may experience physical restrictions caused by their medical condition.

Patients should work with their healthcare professional to develop an exercise program tailored specifically towards taking these limitations into account. Swimming and biking might be better suited than other forms of physical exercise for certain individuals.

Chapter 6: Dialysis Complications and How to Prevent Them

Chapter 6: Dialysis Complications and How to Prevent Them

Complications can arise during dialysis, with potentially harmful results for their health. Here we explore common dialysis complications as well as strategies for how you can avoid them.

1. Hypotension

Hypotension (low blood pressure) is an increasingly prevalent complication during dialysis treatment. If blood pressure drops below normal, patients can experience dizziness, light-headedness, nausea, or fainting, with more serious cases leading to seizures or heart attacks.

Hypotension during dialysis may be caused by several factors: rapid fluid removal, high ultrafiltration rates, autonomic dysfunction, or heart disease. Furthermore, medications like nitroglycerine and alpha-blockers may exacerbate hypotension during dialysis sessions.

How to Avoid Hypotension During Dialysis Slowing the ultrafiltration rate and avoiding too much fluid being removed at once are effective strategies to protect dialysis patients and minimise risks during dialysis sessions. Furthermore, patients should also be instructed to refrain from caffeine, alcohol, and nicotine consumption for several hours before beginning dialysis treatments. Any concurrent use of hypotensive medications may lead to adverse side effects during dialysis sessions.

Prevent dehydration before, during, and after dialysis by regularly monitoring your blood pressure. Interrupt dialysis sessions if hypotension develops.

2. Muscle Cramps

Muscle cramps can be an unpleasant side effect of dialysis treatment, often manifested in leg cramps that cause considerable discomfort for patients. Unfortunately, however, muscle cramps can also impact other muscles throughout the body. Muscle cramps during dialysis remain poorly understood, though various theories for their cause include reduced blood flow from arteriovenous fistula (AVF) closure, electrolyte imbalances, hypotension, dehydration, or nerve sensitivity.

How to Avoid Muscle Cramps while on Dialysis

- Avoid rapid removal of large volumes of fluid.

- Make sure that adequate hydration occurs before,

during, and after dialysis.

- Adjust dialysate calcium concentration according to

individual patient needs.

- Prep muscles before dialysis using heating pads, hot

showers, or stretching exercises.

- Modify the diet and medications of patients suffering

from hypertension, such as increasing magnesium consumption while decreasing phosphate intake and refraining from antihypertensive drugs.

3. Infection

Dialysis patients face an increased risk of infection for various reasons, including reused needles, compromised immune systems, or poor hand hygiene among caregivers.

Infection can strike at any access site - arteriovenous fistula/graft, or bloodstream (sepsis). Signs and symptoms of infection at these two points include fever, chills, warmth, swelling redness and pain at the catheter insertion point or AVF/G site.

How to Avoid Infection During Dialysis Treatment

- Use sterile techniques when accessing the blood vessels of patients.
- Frequently change needle insertion sites and monitor access points for redness, swelling or pain.
- Promote regular hand hygiene practices among both patients and caregivers.
- Use clean and disinfected equipment during dialysis sessions.
- Utilise antimicrobial catheters featuring silver-impregnated cuffs.

4. Anaemia

Dialysis patients frequently develop low red blood cell counts due to end-stage renal disease (ESRD), when their kidneys no longer produce sufficient levels of the erythropoietin hormone that promotes red blood cell production. Coupled with frequent blood loss during dialysis sessions, anaemia quickly sets in.

Anaemia can lead to fatigue, weakness, shortness of breath, decreased cognitive function, and even heart failure if left unchecked. Thus, dialysis patients must monitor and treat anaemia during dialysis treatment to preserve overall health and wellness.

How to Avoid Anaemia During Dialysis
- Monitor haemoglobin levels regularly.

- Add erythropoietin supplements to increase red blood
cell production.
- Administer iron supplements to help build haemoglobin levels.
- Switch your dialysis routines (nocturnal dialysis or
peritoneal) as necessary to decrease blood loss.

5. Dialysis Disequilibrium Syndrome

Dialysis Disequilibrium Syndrome, commonly referred to as DDS, is an uncommon yet severe complication of dialysis that typically impacts newcomers or the severely disabled. DDS occurs when the rapid removal of waste products leads to an excess of blood flow into the brain, which in turn releases water and causes brain swelling.

DDS symptoms include headache, confusion, seizures, tremors, and even comas. Immediate intervention must take place to avoid irreparable brain damage.

6. How to Prevent Dialysis-Delivery System [DDS]

For optimal outcomes, try to avoid rapid removal of large volumes of fluid. Begin with shorter and slower dialysis sessions that increase gradually over time. Increase sodium and protein intake to restore osmotic balance. Monitor patients for any neurological symptoms both during and after dialysis sessions.

By understanding common complications during dialysis treatment, healthcare professionals can take preventative measures to provide optimal care for their patients. Similarly, with proper education and professional guidance, patients can play an active role in minimising or avoiding potential complications during dialysis treatment.

Chapter 7: Strategies for Dealing with Dialysis- Related Fatigue

Chapter 7: Strategies for Dealing with Dialysis- Related Fatigue

Dialysis-related fatigue is a common problem faced by individuals undergoing regular haemodialysis treatment. Fatigue can affect the quality of life among dialysis patients, leading to reduced adherence to treatment and overall health outcomes. Hence, developing strategies to mitigate dialysis-related fatigue is critical for improving the patient's quality of life and treatment outcomes.

Signs and Causes of Dialysis-Related Fatigue

Dialysis-related fatigue is characterised by a feeling of extreme exhaustion that persists even after rest. The causes of dialysis-related fatigue are multi-factorial, and they include anaemia, electrolyte imbalances, malnutrition, fluid overload, sleep disturbances, depression, and inadequate dialysis. Other factors that contribute to fatigue include medication side effects and socio-economic factors. Fatigue can also be a sign of underlying health problems that require medical intervention.

Strategies for Dealing with Dialysis-Related Fatigue

1. Manage Anaemia

Anaemia is a common cause of fatigue in dialysis patients. The lack of erythropoietin production in the kidneys results in reduced red blood cells production, leading to anaemia. Iron supplements are often given to anaemic patients, who have iron-deficiency anaemia, while recombinant

erythropoietin-stimulating agents (ESAs) are used to stimulate the bone marrow to produce red blood cells.

2. Optimise Dialysis Treatment

Inadequate dialysis can also contribute to fatigue symptoms by failing to remove the excess fluid, toxins, and urea from the blood. Dialysis treatment frequency, duration, and intensity must be optimised to achieve adequate clearance to reduce fatigue symptoms. Patients should discuss the possibility of adjusting dialysis prescription with their healthcare providers. Target weight is another factor to consider when optimising dialysis treatments since excess fluid overload can cause fatigue symptoms. Patients must adhere to fluid intake recommendations by monitoring daily fluid intake to avoid fluid overload.

3. **Manage Nutritional Status**

Patients must aim for a well-balanced diet, including proteins, carbohydrates, vitamins, and minerals. Patients should avoid consuming foods that are high in salt, phosphorus, and potassium, which can contribute to electrolyte imbalances and fluid overload. Patients who experience appetite loss can seek the assistance of a dietician to address their nutritional needs. Maintaining proper nutrition can significantly improve energy levels and overall health.

4. **Manage Sleep Disturbances**

Studies show that almost eighty percent of dialysis patients suffer from sleep disorder. Sleep disturbances can lead to exhaustion and contribute to fatigue symptoms. Patients should ensure adequate sleep by acquiring a comfortable

sleeping environment, establishing a regular sleeping schedule, and avoiding daytime napping. Patients must also report to their healthcare provider if they have insomnia or other sleep disorders, as these conditions can be treated with medications and lifestyle interventions.

5. **Address Mental Health**

Depression and anxiety are common among dialysis patients and can contribute to fatigue symptoms. Patients should seek psychological or psychiatric evaluation if they experience symptoms of anxiety or depression. Cognitive behavioural therapy, stress management, or medication can help manage mental health issues and, therefore, improve energy levels and overall well-being.

6. Exercise

Regular exercise is a strategy to manage fatigue among dialysis patients. Engaging in physical activity can help boost energy levels, improve sleep quality, and enhance mood. Patients can start with light exercises, such as walking, stretching, or cycling, and gradually increase intensity and duration. Patients should consult their healthcare providers before engaging in new exercise programs.

7. Supportive Care

Support from family, friends, and support groups can help reduce the feeling of isolation and anxiety that lead to fatigue symptoms. Many dialysis centres and hospitals have support groups that offer emotional and social support to dialysis patients.

Chapter 8: Advocating for Yourself: Tips for Communicating with Healthcare Providers

Chapter 8: Advocating for Yourself: Tips for Communicating with Healthcare Providers

As patients, we rely on healthcare providers to diagnose, treat, and provide guidance for our medical concerns. However, being an informed patient and advocating for yourself can greatly benefit your overall health and well- being. Effective communication with healthcare providers is key to ensuring that you receive high-quality care that aligns with your preferences and values. Here are some tips for communicating with your healthcare providers:

1. Do Your Research Beforehand

Before your appointment, do some research on your symptoms, potential diagnoses, and various treatment options. This will provide you with a foundation of knowledge to build on during your visit, allowing you to ask specific questions and have a more productive conversation with your healthcare provider. Additionally, research the healthcare provider you will be seeing. Knowing their credentials, experience, and specialties can help you better understand their approach to care and how they might be able to assist you.

2. Ask Questions

Don't be afraid to ask your healthcare provider questions. It's important to have a clear understanding of your condition, your treatment options, potential side effects, and any other aspects of your care plan. Openly communicate any concerns or reservations you may have and ask for more information or clarification if needed. Remember, it's your health and your responsibility to advocate for yourself.

3. Be Honest

Honesty is crucial when it comes to discussing your health with your healthcare provider. Be honest about your symptoms, your medical history, and any lifestyle factors that may be affecting your health. Consider sharing information about your job, family life, and other stressors that may be affecting your health. It's also important to let your healthcare provider know if you are not taking your medication as prescribed or if you're experiencing side effects.

4. Bring a Support Person

Having a support person can help you feel more comfortable and confident during your appointment. They can help you remember any questions or concerns you may have, provide emotional support, and advocate for you if needed.

5. Use "I" Statements

Using "I" statements can help you express your concerns and needs more effectively. Instead of saying, "You're taking too long to diagnose me," try saying, "I'm concerned about the length of time it's taking to figure out what's causing my symptoms." This approach can help keep the conversation more positive and productive while still expressing your concerns.

6. Take Notes

It can be helpful to take notes during your appointment to ensure that you don't forget anything important. Write down any recommended treatments, follow-up appointments, or specific instructions. If you don't understand something, don't be afraid to ask your healthcare provider to repeat or explain it again.

7. Follow Up

After your appointment, take time to reflect on the conversation and make sure you understand any next steps in your care plan. If you have additional questions or concerns, don't hesitate to reach out to your healthcare provider. Follow up on recommended treatments or appointments, and don't hesitate to seek a second opinion if needed.

Advocating for yourself as a patient may feel uncomfortable or intimidating but remember that your healthcare providers are there to help you. By being prepared, honest, and open, you can ensure that you receive high-quality care that aligns with your values and preferences.

Chapter 9: Maintaining Relationships

Chapter 9: Maintaining Relationships

When someone is diagnosed with end-stage renal disease (ESRD) and begins dialysis, their life will be significantly impacted. In addition to the physical and emotional toll, dialysis can also affect a person's social life and ability to maintain relationships. Here are some tips for maintaining relationships while on dialysis.

1. Prioritise Communication

Strong communication is essential in any relationship, and this is especially true for those on dialysis. It's important to be open and honest with your loved ones about your condition and the impact it may have on your life.

Communication is key to ensuring that everyone's needs are met and that misunderstandings are avoided. Don't be afraid to talk to your friends and family about your needs and how they can best support you.

2. Consider Talking to a Social Worker

Dialysis centres often have social workers available to help patients and their families navigate the complex emotional and social aspects of living with ESRD. A social worker can provide valuable support and resources, such as counselling, support groups, and community programs. They can also help you connect with others who are going through similar experiences.

3. Join a Support Group

Joining a support group is a great way to connect with others who are going through similar experiences. Support groups can provide a sense of community, emotional support, and a safe space to discuss your concerns. Many dialysis centres offer support groups for patients and their families, and there are also a variety of online support groups and forums available.

4. Continue Participating in Activities You Enjoy

While dialysis may require some lifestyle adjustments, it's important to continue doing the things that bring you joy. Whether it's volunteering, gardening, or attending cultural events, stay involved in activities that make you happy. Finding ways to stay engaged and active can also lead to new social connections and a sense of purpose.

5. Explore Virtual Options

In today's world, virtual options are more prevalent than ever before. Consider joining online communities or social media groups specifically for dialysis patients. Additionally, many dialysis centres offer virtual support groups or activities. These can help you connect with others from the comfort of your own home and offer a sense of community and support.

6. Involve Loved Ones in Your Treatment Plan

While many patients prefer to keep their medical experiences private, involving loved ones in your treatment plan can provide mutual support and strengthen relationships. Consider inviting your family members or close friends to attend a dialysis treatment with you so they can better understand what you are going through.

7. Seek Out Professional Help

Depression, Anxiety, and other mental health conditions are expected effects of dialysis treatment. A mental health professional can provide support and help you develop effective coping strategies for your emotional and psychological needs.

In conclusion, while dialysis can present challenges to relationships and social connections, it is possible to maintain fulfilling connections with loved ones as well as build new relationships. With open communication, involvement of loved ones, and access to support groups and resources, dialysis patients can continue to enjoy active and meaningful social lives. Remember, dialysis is just one aspect of your life – it does not define you or your ability to connect with others.

Chapter 10: Life After Dialysis: Preparing for a Kidney Transplant or End-of-Life Care

Chapter 10: Life After Dialysis: Preparing for a Kidney Transplant or End-of-Life Care

End-stage renal disease (ESRD) can take a significant toll on a person's physical, emotional, and social well-being. Dialysis is a common treatment option for individuals with ESRD, but it is often not a permanent solution. Many patients begin to consider their options for life after dialysis, including kidney transplants and end-of-life care. Here are some tips for preparing for both options.

Kidney Transplant

1. Explore Your Options

The first step in preparing for a kidney transplant is to explore your options. You can discuss with your healthcare provider, dialysis treatment team, or a kidney specialist about your eligibility for a transplant, the transplantation process, and the risks and benefits associated with it. They can also help you find a transplant centre and connect you with transplant surgeons to evaluate your eligibility.

2. Get on the Transplant Waitlist

If you are eligible for a kidney transplant, the next step is to get on the transplant waitlist. This involves contacting a nearby transplant centre and undergoing an evaluation to determine your eligibility. If you are determined to be a suitable candidate, you will be placed on the waitlist until a kidney donor becomes available.

3. Consider Living Donation

Living donation is a process where a healthy person donates one of their kidneys to someone in need. The wait time for a kidney from a living donor is typically shorter than for a deceased donor, and the success rates of living donor transplants are typically higher. Consider reaching out to family members and close friends to see if anyone is willing to be a living donor. Alternatively, you can also consider the paired exchange programs to where your donor may not compatible with you, but they find a matched with another individual who has a compatible donor kidney to you.

4. Prepare for Surgery and Recovery

If you are fortunate enough to find a donor or they select you for a deceased donor transplant, it's crucial to prepare for surgery and the recovery period. This may involve arranging transportation to and from the transplant centre, ensuring that you have a supportive care team, and making any necessary lifestyle changes prior to surgery. You'll also need to commit to post-transplant care, including taking immunosuppressive medication, which can reduce the likelihood of organ rejection but can pose additional risks to your health.

End-of-Life Care

1. Make Your Wishes Known

Preparing for end-of-life care can be daunting, but it is an important consideration. Living wills, advanced care directives, and healthcare proxies are all legal documents that can help ensure that your wishes regarding medical care, life support, and end-of-life care are respected. Discuss your wishes with your healthcare team and family members to ensure they fully understand what you want.

2. Connect with Hospice and Palliative Care Services

If you decide to forgo further dialysis treatment, hospice and palliative care services can provide comfort care and support for you and your loved ones during the end-of-life process. Hospice care can provide pain management, symptom relief, and emotional support, while palliative care can help manage your symptoms and improve your quality of life.

3. Seek Emotional Support

Dealing with a life-limiting illness can take a significant emotional toll on you and your loved ones. Consider seeking emotional support from a therapist, social worker, or support group. They can help you work through your emotions, deal with grief or anxiety, and connect with others who are going through similar experiences.

4. Plan Funeral Arrangements

Planning funeral arrangements can help ease the burden on your loved ones during an already difficult time. You can discuss your preferences for a funeral or memorial service with your family members and make arrangements for final resting places. Financial planning for a funeral or memorial service is also a vital step.

In conclusion, preparing for life after dialysis can be challenging but important. Whether you decide to pursue a kidney transplant or focus on end-of-life care, there are steps you can take to prepare yourself and your loved ones for the road ahead. By exploring your options, making your wishes known, seeking support, and planning ahead, you can take control of your health and ensure that your needs are met.

BIBLIOGRAPHY

1. KIDNEY DIALYSIS: Understand The Complete Process Of Dialysis With A Step By Step Guide Into The Process, Benefits, Disadvantages And More For Beginners by Judge Brown -2022

2. Renal Diet: The Complete Nutrition Guide to Manage Kidney Disease, and Avoiding Dialysis. Delicious Recipes Low Sodium, Low Phosphorus and Low Potassium for Healthy Kidney by Cristina Collins -2020

3. Dialysis without Fear: A Guide to Living Well on Dialysis for Patients and Their Families:- by Daniel Offer, Marjorie Kaiz Offer and Susan Offer Szafir-2007

4. Psychosocial Aspects of End-Stage Renal Disease: Issues of Our Times by Elizabeth Clark-1991

5. Nutritional and Pharmacological Strategies in Chronic Renal Failure by A. Albertazzi, P. Cappelli and G. Del Rosso-1991

More About Author

In 2010, Lord M. A. Daley Sr. received a rare kidney disease diagnosis called C1Q Nephropathy at the age of thirty-five, despite no prior history of renal disease within his family. From 2012, he has been undergoing haemodialysis as a patient at the Basingstoke Dialysis Unit. A failed kidney transplant resulted from the aggressive nature of his rare renal disease in 2014. After thoughtful consideration, Lord Daley decided to continue with dialysis treatment. His proactive approach towards healthcare is evident in his advice to other patients, which encourages taking responsibility for one's well-being.

Printed in Great Britain
by Amazon